Say Hello to an Acne-Free You

How to Cure Acne and Keep It from Coming Back

By: Janet Crawford

9781681275123

PUBLISHERS NOTES

Disclaimer – Speedy Publishing LLC

This publication is intended to provide helpful and informative material. It is not intended to diagnose, treat, cure, or prevent any health problem or condition, nor is intended to replace the advice of a physician. No action should be taken solely on the contents of this book. Always consult your physician or qualified health-care professional on any matters regarding your health and before adopting any suggestions in this book or drawing inferences from it.

The author and publisher specifically disclaim all responsibility for any liability, loss or risk, personal or otherwise, which is incurred as a consequence, directly or indirectly, from the use or application of any contents of this book.

Any and all product names referenced within this book are the trademarks of their respective owners. None of these owners have sponsored, authorized, endorsed, or approved this book.

Always read all information provided by the manufacturers' product labels before using their products. The author and publisher are not responsible for claims made by manufacturers.

This book was originally printed before 2014. This is an adapted reprint by Speedy Publishing LLC with newly updated content designed to help readers with much more accurate and timely information and data.

Speedy Publishing LLC

40 E Main Street, Newark, Delaware, 19711

Contact Us: 1-888-248-4521

Website: http://www.speedypublishing.co

REPRINTED Paperback Edition: 9781681275123:

Manufactured in the United States of America

DEDICATION

This book is dedicated to Nathan. You are the little guy I have loved even without having met you yet.

TABLE OF CONTENTS

Chapter 1- Are Those Red Marks on Your Skin Acne?

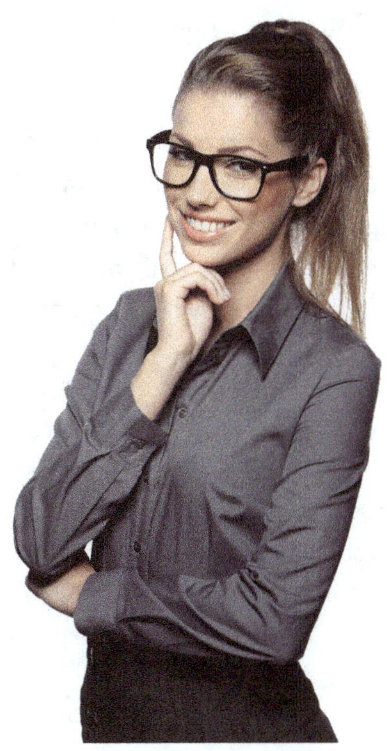

Acne is a disease in which the hair follicles on your skin become clogged and infected. This results in one of the three types of acne lesions to form.

The production of excess sebum is the culprit. It causes the follicles to become blocked. The medical community is still uncertain as to what triggers this excess production. Sebum is produced by the sebaceous oil gland and everybody needs a small amount to achieve healthy skin. Sebum helps protects the skin from harmful bacteria by washing it away.

Types of Acne Lesions

The three types of acne lesions are whiteheads & blackheads (also known as closed and open comedones respectively), papules & pustules, and cysts.

Whiteheads as the name suggests, look like white bumps. They form under the skin and never reach the surface. This makes them very hard to eliminate. Blackheads grow upward and break the skins surface. This enlarged follicle and the oxidation of the dead cells, sebum, and bacteria have a black color, hence the name.

Papules form when a whitehead burst and the bacteria spreads to the surrounding tissues under the skin. This causes your body's immune system to increase its fight on the infection making the inflammation worse. They appear as small, firm, red bumps. Pustules form as the body's immune system continues to fight the infection by sending pus to the area. They appear similar to papules with the addition of a yellowish white head.

Cysts are the third and final type of acne lesion. They form when a pustule worsens and expands further down under the skins surface. They appear red or purple and are very painful. This is the most serious of all types of acne lesions.

Types of Acne

Acne can not only be classified by the types of acne lesions, but further broken down by acne type; depending on what types of lesions you have. People whose acne consists of whiteheads and blackheads would have what is called comedonal acne. A mix of blackheads, whiteheads, papules and pustules acne lesions is called acne vulgaris and is the most common type of acne. The third type of acne is called cystic acne and it is when someone has all three types of acne lesions with numerous cysts.

Who Can Get Acne?

While most people associate acne with teens, anybody can experience some type of acne at any age. That said certain groups of people are more likely to experience acne. They include teens, people under stress, people who have a family history of the disease, people taking certain drugs and adult women.

What Causes Acne?

Acne begins in puberty, but it does not always end there. Every teenager, if examined closely enough will show some of the effects of acne with some being mild, others more severe. The major hormone causing changes in teenagers is androgen. Under its influence, the sebaceous glands produce more and more sebum (oil). This leads, then, to oily skin and a change in skin flora. There is an increase in the bacteria that cause acne as well as a type of fungus. All these contribute to the development of blockages at the oil gland openings known as comedones. Such blockages cause blackheads and whiteheads – and acne when there is infection of the skin's pores.

Acne should not be viewed as something that comes with puberty. It has lasting effects on the skin, like scarring, and should be treated. A gentle skin cleansing without using cleansers that over-dry skin should be established. Addition to that a supplement such as Acuzine should be taken to have a fast and effective acne cure inside out.

In adults, acne could be a carryover from adolescence, occupational (exposure to chemicals or other skin irritants in the workplace), drug induced (some medications exacerbate acne) or cosmetic acne. There are also other factors that may contribute to acne besides family history such as frequent use of thick make-up, frequent activities under hot and humid conditions and contact with oily substances.

There is nothing much that we can do about genetics but surely we can do something about lifestyle factors to prevent acne. Using thick, oily creams also may lead to breakouts too. People with acne should use products that are formulated for people with oily skin.

Stress is another common aggravating factor for acne. Lack of sleep is a form of stress in itself too. And for women, the menstrual cycle can trigger off acne too. But whatever your stage in life with acne, if the acne cream or lotion show no sign of clearing up, then get Acuzine. Acuzine is rate no.1 acne treatment product with guaranteed results. It works for adults or teenagers suffering from facial or body acne. This is a natural acne treatment formula with no side effect and highly recommended by dermatologists. Fast and effective acne cure from inside out.

• Masturbation or sex

Sex or masturbation does not cause acne. Studies done to relate sex or masturbation to acne are inconclusive with no additional evidence. An old wives' tale, this acne myth became popular during the early 17th century to discourage women from engaging in pre-marital sex or other scandalous behavior. Some misleading adults even use the fear of having acne to discourage adolescents of today from engaging in sex at an early age.

• Chocolates and oily food

Although eating too much of sweets and oily food is never good for anybody, the relationship between acne and this food group is largely indirect. Hormonal changes, which are the most common cause of acne, may cause a person to alternately crave sweet and salty food like chocolates and chips. Since this craving often coincides with acne flare ups, this food group has been misleadingly labeled as a cause of acne.

Treating acne at the start of the problem is easier than dealing with the scars.

Is It True That Adults Get Acne When They Reach 30?

Adult acne is a form of common acne that can occur to people over 30 years of age. It is not uncommon for people who had no acne as a young person to found that they are having breakouts.

Acne appearance in an adult could have a number of causes.

The following are seven causes of adult acne:

1. Frequently the acne that one had as a teenager resurfaces later in adulthood. It is not always obvious why this occurs, but it is one reason for acne presence in adults.

2. In women, acne often reappears during pregnancy. This could also be true in the case of women during their menstrual period.

3. Something unusual is going on. It is smart idea to talk to a dermatologist or your family physician.

More possible causes of adult acne:

4. Particular medications can provoke acne. These medications include anabolic steroids, lithium, anti-tuberculosis drugs rifampin and isoniazid, anti-epileptic drugs and medications that contain iodine.

5. Constant physical pressure on the skin. Wearing a helmet or carrying a backpack can cause breakouts.

6. Chlorinated industrial chemicals are another possible cause. Working in particular types of industrial environments can cause acne-like symptoms or even chloracne - a job-related skin disorder caused by constant exposure to chemicals, such as chlorinated dioxins.

7. Metabolic changes are yet another cause of adult acne. Changes in the hormonal balance of the body like during menstruation or pregnancy can cause acne in adults.

Should You Be Concerned About Baby Acne?

Small babies may develop acne because of the lingering maternal hormones after delivery, which may cause stimulation to the baby's sebaceous glands. Your baby receives these hormones from the placenta, after the delivery.

Don't worry if your baby has pimples. About 20% of the newborn babies are affected by baby acne, also known as acne-neonatorum.

Let' know the various aspects of this peculiar type of acne. First things first, the treatment for infantile acne is not the same as that of acne treatment for any other age group.

Infantile acne is gender-biased. Male babies are more affected than their female counterparts. Normally babies have the acne attack at the age of 3 weeks. Some babies have it from the time of delivery. Generally the types of acne you find in infants are papules and pustules. Papules are red bumps and pustules are whiteheads. They have a collection of pus.

Some babies also have acne on the scalp. Acne in babies does not require treatment as such. The lesions will take care of themselves within a period of four months. But do take the normal care of the baby as you would take care of its other body parts.

Use mild baby soap and gently clean the face once in a day with water. Do not try harsher methods by using oil and other lotions which you think are good. They may at times, worsen the condition. Know for certain that infantile acne will disappear when it has to.

In your anxiety to photograph the baby, don't stuff his/her cheeks with cosmetics and if at all you need to have the touch-ups, do it in an imaginative way.

If you or your family doctor feels that the baby has severe acne, treat it with benzoyl peroxide, keratolytic agents or topical creams like retinoids.

The ways of acne are indeed mysterious. If you have a family history of acne, that doesn't mean that your baby will have acne. And just because the baby has acne, it doesn't mean that, it will suffer from the attack of acne, when it grows up. Acne has its own working style and attacking strategy.

Infantile acne, which normally appears after the age of three months in a baby, quietly disappears after the age of 12 months.

Say Hello to an Acne-Free You
No special efforts of treatment are required. In some babies, the condition may last up to three years. It is due to the genetic makeup of your baby. You have something to contribute to it, as the hereditary part.

You have nothing to do with the infantile acne, relating to the treatment part. Just observe its arrival and departure. Well, arrival with anxiety and departure with pleasure!

CHAPTER 2- PREVENTING BREAKOUTS

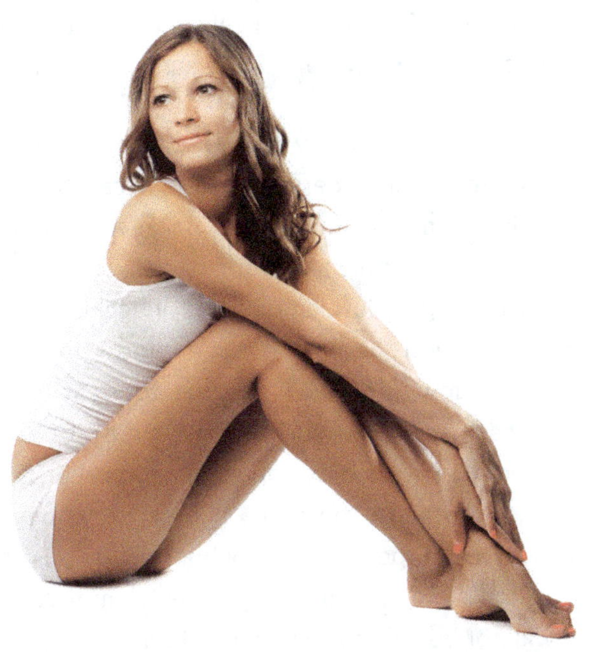

Back acne comes in all sizes and forms of acne, ranging from mild forms like whiteheads to serious forms of acne including cystic acne. "Bacne" as it is referred to in slang terms, can consist of pimples, pustules and blackheads as well. Back acne affects people ranging from age ten to age forty or older yet. Understanding the causes of back acne and available treatment options, are very important is treating and preventing the condition.

Like all of the other forms of acne, there is no one thing that causes back acne. As far as the medical community stands, back acne also happens when oil glands start functioning more rapidly around puberty. The hormone group androgens, found in both females and males, get overactive which in turn causes a reaction in the oil glands, which make extra oil. The oil glands are located just underneath the skin surface. Oil glands constantly are producing and secreting oil through the pores in the skin. When too much of the oils are produced the pores and hair follicles become clogged. The clogs obstruct the way that dead cells escape the skin, which in turn results in a mess of oil and dead cells plugging the hair follicle. This attracts bacterium, which causes the acne to be formed.

Back acne can be found on any part of the body and does not necessarily have to be on a person's back. It can be very severe with large lesions and painful cysts. Back acne may just be something that certain people are prone to or it could be caused by other things such as tight clothing or a heavy backpack. Not having anything in contact with the back is not a logical prevention step, as we all must sit down and everyone has to wear clothing. It is easier to treat back acne than to try and prevent it because most people suffer from back acne at one time or another. Skin on the back is much thicker and therefore allows for stronger topical treatments, such as ten percent Benzoyl peroxide. This strength of Benzoyl peroxide is not suitable for other skin that is typically thinner and will not be able to sustain itself under harsh treatment. You can get all the same types of acne, blackheads, whiteheads, papules, pustules and cysts, on your back just as you can on any other part of your body.

There are some differences in back acne and acne located elsewhere on the body however. Back acne is not caused by genetics as other acnes can be. Some severe cases of back acne may be genetically passed on but most likely it is just the individual's body type or personal genetic make-up. People all over the world suffer from back acne at some point in their lives. Unlike other acne, food does not contribute to the formation or flare up of back acne. There is absolutely no evidence that foods cooked in grease, or high in fat content contribute to back acne.

It is also known that excessive oil production and dirt build up does not have a huge impact on developing back acne. Perspiring excessively and not washing or showering immediately has been shown to not increase the chances of developing back acne. Back acne also does not seem to be affected by stress. There are some who think that facial acne is increased due to stress. However stress can cause back acne to not heal. Oftentimes, stress causes people to pick and bother the pimples, which make the condition worse.

Taking some over the counter medicines may treat breakouts of back acne in conditions that are not complex. Some skin specialists or dermatologists should treat severe forms of acne on the back, such as cystic acne. Most of the simpler forms of acne might disappear with daily washing and cleansing routines but as cystic acne goes deep into the skin and can cause permanent scarring, it should be given more serious medical attention than simple pustules or blackheads on the back. Always speak to your healthcare provider about treatment before starting a back acne treatment program never attempt to treat severe acne on your own or with an over the counter product without consulting a professional.

Seasonal Breakouts

Acne, one of the most common skin conditions, affects more than four out of five people between the ages of 12 and 24. With summer and wedding season under way, you may want to learn more about acne by seeing if you know the correct answers to these commonly asked questions:

Q. Will frequent face washing eliminate acne?

A. Although a popular belief, dirty skin does not cause acne, and frequent face washing and scrubbing can actually make acne worse.

Q. Is acne caused by poor nutritional choices?

A. Scientific studies have not found a clear link between diet and acne. In other words, chocolate or greasy foods do not cause or worsen acne in most people. If acne is being treated appropriately, there's no need to worry about certain foods leading to a breakout.

Q. Will squeezing pimples make them go away quicker?

A. No. It is recommended that those with acne avoid squeezing, pinching or picking at the face. Any sort of skin friction created by rubbing or leaning can actually make acne worse.

Q. Is acne just part of adolescence?

A. Although many teens are affected by acne, it is important to know that acne may be improved with proper treatment. Teens with acne should see a family doctor or dermatologist for the appropriate treatment. Acne that is not treated may lead to permanent physical scars, which can affect how people feel about themselves.

Q. Are all acne medications the same?

A. No. There is a wide range of over-the-counter (OTC) and prescription medications that can be used to help treat acne. Some medications help reduce the buildup of too much oil and fight bacteria associated with pimples; other medications help unclog the pores. The number-one prescribed combination acne product in the U.S. is BenzaClin® (clindamycin 1 percent-benzoyl peroxide 5 percent gel), a combination of benzoyl peroxide and clindamycin that helps fight bacteria and reduces inflammation of pimples. Because acne varies from patient to patient, it is important that people with acne consult their physician to find out which type of treatment is best for them.

It is important to know that acne may be improved with treatment and those suffering from it can do something about it.

What's the Worst That Can Happen?

Severe acne can cause physical as well as emotional scars. Although most people stress out over the occasional zit, acne can deliver serious blows to an individual's sense of confidence and self-perception. Acne can cause a person to experience consistently blemished skin that may include pimples, papules, abscesses, cysts, blackheads, whiteheads, and other painful inflammations of the skin. Moreover, acne can be a whole body problem. While most people are seriously afflicted primarily in the facial area, many people also experience considerable blemishing across their back, chest, neck, and other areas of the body.

While most people experience the brunt of acne during the difficult adolescent years, imagine the agony of living with acne well into your middle years. With the stress of modern day living and increased exposure to environmental pollutants, adult acne is becoming a fact of life for many adults. Although most people will only have to deal with transient acne, some will experience far worse. Here is a quick run-down of the most serious forms of acne.

Acne Conglobata (AC) - This is a very uncommon form of acne that can produce significant disfiguration. Acne conglobata is characterized by the development of burrows in the skin, along with papules, abscesses, keloidal and atrophic facial scars. Individuals with AC often develop blemishes that appear in clusters of two or three. Cysts are often present that are filled with pus. Nodules may also be present, especially in the area of the back and chest.

Who is more susceptible to acne conglobata? In general, males are more likely to experience AC. Onset of AC usually occurs at a young age, between the ages of 18 and 30. Although no one knows the exact cause of AC, some believe it is caused by a mutation in the XXY karyotype chromosomes. A person with AC may experience extensive scarring and subsequent disfigurement. Because the effects of AC can often be dramatic, individuals afflicted with the skin disorder may be at greater risk of suffering from self-esteem issues, depression, anxiety, and they may feel stigmatized.

Acne Fulminans (AF): Acne fulminans, sometimes referred to as acne maligna, was originally thought to be acne conglobata (AC).

The major characteristics of acne fulminans include sudden onset of ulcerating acne, which may be accompanied by fever and symptoms of polyarthritis. Usually, AF does not respond well to conventional acne treatment, such as antibacterial therapy. The most successful treatments appear to be debridement used in conjunction with steroid therapy.

What causes AF? It appears that acne fulminans is caused by a weakened immune system and increased levels of testosterone and certain anabolic steroids. These high levels of hormones cause an increase in the production and excretion of sebum and the acne-inducing bacteria known as propionibacterium acnes (P acnes). Some skin professionals believe that isotretinoin may also precipitate an eruption of AF.

How can you tell the difference between acne conglobata and acne fulminans? Although the physical symptoms may at first appear identical, AF is usually characterized by the presence of more physical pain. Patients with AF may describe feelings of bone or facial pain, migraines, and fever. Acne conglobata and acne fulminans also differ in the way they are treated. While AC may be treated with conventional anti-acne oral and topical agents, AF typically does not respond well to such treatments. AF responds better to steroid treatments.

Gram-Negative Folliculitis: Gram-negative folliculitis refers to an infection of gram-negative rods that usually occurs after an extended period of antibiotic therapy. Scientists use the word "gram" to describe the blue stain that is used in laboratories. This is often used to locate microscopic organisms. The bacteria that cause gram-negative folliculitis does not stain blue, thus the term 'gram-negative.' The most common forms of bacteria that are believed to cause gram-negative folliculitis include E. coli, serratia marcesoens, pseudomonas aeruginosa, and bacteria's from the proteus and klebsiella species.

How does gram-negative folliculitis differ from regular acne vulgaris? Most cases of gram-negative folliculitis produce less papules and comedones than acne vulgaris. Treatment of gram-negative folliculitis is fortunately much easier to treat than other severe types of acne. In most cases, conventional antibiotic therapy will help clear up gram-negative folliculitis. Isotretinoin may also help clear up this condition.

Chapter 3- Can a Change in Diet Eliminate Acne?

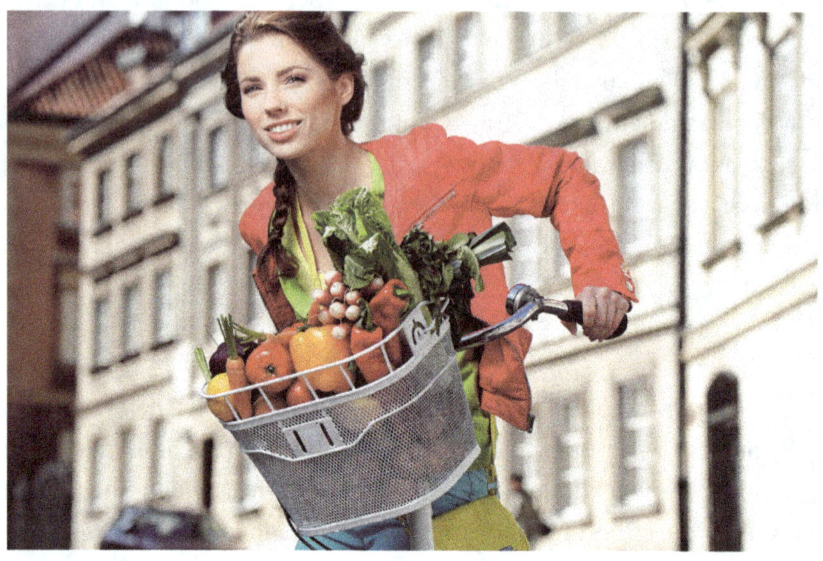

Acne, as you may notice, affects additional than ninety percent of the world's population at some occasion in their life. It is in detail the most common skin disease treated by dermatologist and most of its victims are teenagers and adults. According to some technical research, acne is caused by different factors like hormones, bacteria, and some genetic factors. Some even oral that acne is caused by a poor diet, to which many did not agree.

Well, the acne and diet issue has been studied for several years. Although some dermatologist claimed that diet has naught to do with the formation of acne, many still hold that acne and diet has a certain dovetail. Acne and diet are somehow correlated as diet plays a role in the maturation of acne. Here's a common interpretation that cede show how acne and diet are connected.

Certain studies own found out that eating pure carbohydrates and sugar leads to a surge of insulin as well as an insulin - like swelling factor proclaimed as IGF - 1 in the article. If this forms, it then can escort to an excess of mainly hormones, androgens, which are deemed as the most potent produce of the acne formation. The acne and diet connection maintains that if an excess of manlike hormones is produced, the pores of the skin leave emit sebum or oil, which is a greasy substance that generally pulls the weight of acne - causing bacteria. In addendum, this process triggers the IGF - 1 to create skin cells proclaimed as keratinocytes to duplicate and multiply, which in turn is a process material with the acne formation.

Further, the dovetail between acne and diet is shown with the impact of certain studies conducted on the acne cases in islanders of Papua New Guinea and hunter - gatherers of Paraguay. According to this acne and diet connection study, the face of acne is triggered by some environmental factors to which diet is one. Many possess found out through such acne and diet study that limiting grains is an integral pace toward optimizing your health, which led the researchers to think that no - grain diet is somehow salutary for acne.

Today, the acne and diet fit is one of the hottest issues in the medical field. Many own claimed that there is only little research regarding the connection between acne and diet for there is no money in it. Some even claimed that doctors and dermatologists only chat that diet has naught to do with acne since they can't sell you a healthy diet. Now, come to think of it, underneath it all, acne just like some diseases is caused by diet, but you can't cure it by just focusing on the diet since some other aggravators are behind it.

Adding Vitamins A and E Might Help

In the fight against acne, vitamins A and E both act fairly similarly and both have great advantages for preventing its outbreak. Needless to say, getting proper amounts of these vitamins into your body every day is crucial for maintaining clear, healthy skin and for helping to prevent acne from becoming a problem.

Vitamin A fights acne initially by helping to strengthen the protective tissue of the skin. Additionally, it reduces sebum (oil) production in the skin. This combination helps the skin to become more capable of fighting acne and also this healthy skin, with less oil, is less likely to suffer from acne breakouts. Furthermore, Vitamin A is a very strong antioxidant which helps to rid the body, including the skin, of harmful toxins and free radicals, therefore helping to clear the skin of many problems, including acne. Vitamin A is usually taken in conjunction with carotenoids which enhances its effects against acne.

Vitamin E is also an antioxidant. Although not as strong of one as Vitamin A, Vitamin E still does help to rid the skin of toxins which can lead to acne and helps to clear up existing acne. Vitamin E also promotes tissue repair and healing of the skin, two important aspects that help to both strengthen the skin and also to prevent damage caused by acne to become permanent. Additionally, Vitamin E prevents cell damage by inhibiting the oxidation of lipids (fats) and the formation of free radicals.

As can be seen, both vitamins have fairly similar methods of assisting in the fight against acne. Both help to strengthen the skin and healthier, stronger skin is less prone to acne. Both are also antioxidants and help to clear the skin of acne and prevent future breakouts. The difference is that Vitamin A reduces oil production and Vitamin E promotes tissue repair and healing. In combination, these vitamins are extremely effective in combating acne.

Both Vitamin A and Vitamin E are extremely important vitamins and a deficiency in either of them can lead to acne. Consuming healthy amounts of these vitamins every day can help to fight existing acne and also to enable to body to better prevent further acne breakouts from occurring. Put plainly, both of these vitamins should be involved in any methods used to combat acne and should be heavily considered when looking for acne fighting vitamin supplements.

Chapter 4- Common Acne Treatments

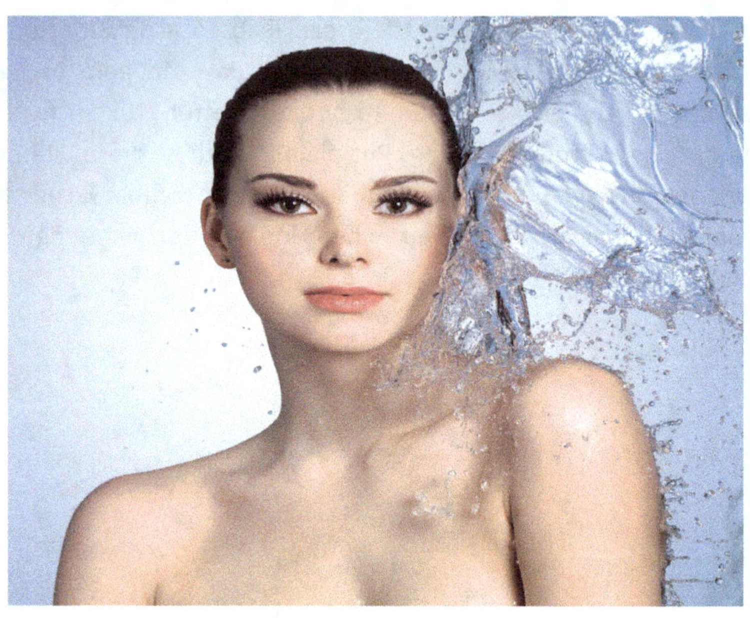

Acne treatment has many varieties. Acne is a broad term which includes blemishes, blackheads, and whiteheads. See acne information for more. Acne can strike at any age. Effective acne treatment is sometimes difficult to find, and understanding acne and prevention can be frustrating. Below are some acne treatment tips that have worked for many. Understanding acne treatment is a very important step to take before undergoing the treatment itself.

Although acne isn't life threatening it can be uncomfortable and hard on your ego. There has always been a debate about the actual cause of acne. The actual cause isn't as important as finding a cure. There's acne treatment for teenagers that has been specifically configured for the teenage age group. Adult acne is also common and adults can experience acne problems well into their 40's.

So is there a cure for acne? Well yes and no. There are many products available and for some they are a cure, for others they do not help. A cure is only a cure when you find a product that works for you.

Most acne treatments will take time to work. It usually takes around 8 weeks before you see any significant improvement so you are going to have to be patient. Once your acne's cleared up it's important to continue with the acne treatment that's working so it does not return.

If you have serious acne it is best to consult a dermatologist. However in milder cases you will often be able to get it under control by yourself just by persevering. Try these acne treatment tips to conquer your acne.

• Acne control through exercise

Regular exercise helps keep your whole body in shape. It builds your immune system and helps eliminate toxins from the body. It's a great start to fighting acne.

• Diet can act as acne medicine

You need to eat at least 5 servings of fresh fruit and vegetables each day. Fresh fruit and vegetables are full of nutrients that your body needs. They boost the immune system and are good antioxidants. They can work towards helping you get rid of the acne. Try to avoid refined sugars and fatty foods which have are not good for you or your skin. You also need to drink at least 8 glasses of water a day to flush your system of toxins.

• Cosmetics can help acne treatment

Choose cosmetics that are water based and hypo-allergenic. Avoid oil free products, coal tar derivatives, and heavy creams. Make sure you wash your skin thoroughly every night to remove makeup residue.

• Hormones and acne

Hormones can play a role in acne flare ups and they can be used to reduce outbreaks. Your doctor may decide to use HRT to eliminate or reduce your acne outbreaks.

• Clean skin for acne treatment

You need to avoid harsh scrubbing of your face but you also need to thoroughly clean your skin nightly. Use a mild cleaning regime every night. Once or twice a week use an exfoliator to gently remove damaged skin and unplug pores. Also see acne skin care tips that work.

• Shaving and acne

Is actually a great exfoliating treatment the removes dead skin. However you should never shave an area that is infected or inflamed. Always use a shaving cream if your skin is sensitive.

• Stress and acne control

Can be a contributing factor to acne so try to relax and unwind. Emotions trigger chemical reactions in the body which can cause an outbreak.

You can help control your acne outbreaks by following these simple steps.

Natural Alternatives

Although most of the dermatologists disregard the importance of healthy diet for a healthy skin as diet lacking vital supplements is scientifically proven not to affect the skin quality in any way, but there are some diets that tone the skin and make it healthy.

The first step of herbal acne treatment should be making sure that your diet contains enough fatty acid foods and foods that are the source of multi-vitamins.

Features of Herbal Acne Treatment Products

Herbal acne treatment products are famous for their following features.

• Noticeable improvement in acne condition within one week

• Complete removal of acne within three weeks

• Elimination of acne scars

• Inclusion of herbs that beautify the skin after the disappearance of acne and the scars

• All the above benefits with virtually no side-effects

• Affordability

Herbs in Herbal Acne Treatment Products

Following herbs are commonly included in herbal acne treatment products.

Rose Hips:

Rose Hips or Rosa Affinis Rubiginosa in herbal acne treatment products provide rejuvenation to dry and aging skin. It is also a proven cure for acne.

Lemongrass:

Lemongrass or Cymbopogon Citratus is the herb many herbal acne treatment products contain due to its capability to calm acne.

Chamomile:

Chamomile or Matricaria Recutita helps soothes sensitive skin and is commonly found in many hot-selling herbal acne treatment products.

Rosemary:

Rosemary or Rosmarinus Officinalis is another herb that is included in the best rated herbal acne treatment products. This herb is known for its capability to stimulate and protect skin. This is also famous for its acne healing effects.

Can You Make Acne Treatments from Home?

The difference between natural acne treatments products and non-natural acne treatment products is that difference except natural treatment products does not include any side effects. Although natural acne treatment products have been increasing its popularity over the latest few years, another popular type of acne treatment was found, the home made acne treatment products.

Homemade acne treatment products may range from natural products to non-natural products. The greatest advantage is that one can use different acne treatment products until you find one that they prefer and that works best on them. So this way they do not need to buy many different products to find one that works best but easily make the product at home to try it and then make more when it gives a good result.

Still sometimes these treatment products can be natural; they also give the advantages of natural treatment products, no side effects. They are still acne treatment products but they may take longer to treat the acne, sometimes it may take up to months with a homemade acne treatment product to make the acne go away.

Basically homemade acne treatments are made with the sources that one has. Since everyone is different, the identical acne treatment product will not give the same results to everyone. Therefore homemade acne treatment can quickly find the perfect acne treatment product for you. This type of acne treatment has been gaining popularity for a long time now. This type of acne treatment is also the cheapest kind of acne treatment out there. Some researchers have found that other people's remedies for acne will not work sometimes but then when using a homemade acne remedy; it could do the job and get rid of your acne.

There is also one bad point in using homemade acne treatments. They might not work and may sometimes add to the problem. If the treatment has not been made correctly it may add to the acne problem with side effects and other skin issues. Most people would just use trial and error because most of the skin issues that is caused by a side effect can be cured. It is best to do some research before making your own home made acne treatment product.

Acne Treatment Myths

We'll just come out and say it; there is a lot of misleading and downright wrong information out there about acne. Thankfully, scientific research has dispelled a lot of these 'acne myths'. We now have a pretty good idea of what does and does not cause acne. Let's take a look at seven of the biggest of these acne myths.

True or False? Find out the truth about common acne and its myths

Acne Myth #1: Acne is caused by eating certain foods

This one has been around a long time yet is supported by exactly no scientific proof. Although certain individuals may seem experience outbreaks when they eat certain foods, there are no universal laws that apply to everyone. Eating pizza, chocolate, nuts, and greasy foods will not increase your acne.

Acne Myth #2: Acne is related to dirt or having dirty skin

Although having clean skin has other benefits, dirt does not cause acne. Acne is formed under the surface of the skin and is due to build-ups of sebum and dead skin cells. It's not dirt that clogs your follicles.

Acne Myth #3: Washing your face all the time will clear up acne

This kind of relates to myth #3. Having clean skin is not the answer to preventing acne. Overdoing it as far as washing your face can actually make matters worse. Stripping your skin of oil could lead to future breakouts.

Acne Myth #4: Only teenagers get acne

It is true that 9 out of 10 teenagers experience acne, but it is also true that about 1 in 4 adults get it also. Acne seems to be connected with hormones which would explain why teenagers have such a high incidence of acne, but adults are also going through hormonal changes at various times in their lives.

Acne Myth #5: Stress causes acne

Scientific evidence shows that stress is not that large of a factor in acne. It was believed for many years that stress caused bouts of acne but it simply isn't so.

Acne Myth # 6: Acne can be cured

Many people view acne as a disease that can be permanently cured. Unfortunately, this isn't the case. Acne can be controlled and prevented through proper skin care, but it cannot be cured.

Treatment Get More Complicated with Adult Acne

People who are suffering with mild to severe adult acne can be treated with tropical or oral medicines. The main aim of any best adult acne treatment should include prevention of scarring and clearance of acne. For severe form of adult acne systemic therapy is mainly used. Remember not every popular adult acne products work well for everyone. The exact reasons for adult acne is unknown but is believed to relate to the changes or imbalance in an individual's body hormones.

Treatment

Acne is the most common skin affliction in the world, yet quality acne treatment is still a mystery to many sufferers. The main aim of any best adult acne treatment should include prevention of scarring and clearance of acne. Most people who suffer from acne go out and spend good money on common over-the-counter acne treatment products.

See what others have to say about specific acne treatment products before you buy them. This is a major factor to consider when searching for acne treatment products. There are infinite acne treatment products on the market today. If you jump online, you will notice a great variety of acne treatment products with numerous reviews to boot. Most people who suffer from acne go out and spend good money on common over-the-counter acne treatment products.

Experts suggest that you never use standard bath soap. Next on your list of cystic acne treatments is a face moisturizer. Ex-acne sufferer reveals what natural acne cures work, what acne treatments to avoid, and more surprising acne information. I have been through all sorts of acne treatments, including Accutane multiple times, and Proactiv was very effective for me! It is the most effective and easy-to-use product that I have encountered in my search for acne treatments.

For some the cheapest acne products do the job, for others it is the most expensive. To get the best out of any over the counter acne products you need to use them consistently and correctly. Remember not every popular adult acne products work well for everyone.

Treating Mild Acne

Acne has three stages of diseases - mild, moderate and severe. If acne can be treated during the first stage itself, you can save tremendous amount of effort and protect yourself from the agony of bad looking scars that form after third stage of acne. Catch acne in the mild stage itself and do not let it grow to second and third stage.

Mild acne does not need more intensive forms of treatment. Many acne sufferers treat themselves with OTC medicines for acne. Some patients prefer to consult a doctor at this stage itself to protect them from any flare up of acne.

Let us discuss the common treatment available for mild acne. Over the counter medications consisting of salicylic acid or benzoyl peroxide can control mild acne that is mainly whiteheads and blackheads. While using these medications, wash your acne prone area with mild sop/cleanser and warm water twice a day to remove excess oil and dead skin.

Sometimes these products may cause dryness, redness or peeling. Use an oil free moisturizer if the peeling is present. The skin takes some time to adjust to the acne medication. If irritation occurs, you should consult your doctor. Please remember that acne medication takes time to treat acne. Many time up to eight weeks to work. Keep patience and wait for the results to get acne cured. If you do not get results after that, you should consult your doctor. Your doctor may prescribe other medicines to treat acne.

Testing the Blue Light to Treat Acne

Some experts claim that laser and light therapy is this century's alternative to traditional treatments. These technologies have been successfully applied to treating acne and other skin diseases. Many acne sufferers who were disappointed with all other methods have found a solution for their problem in blue light acne treatment.

Benefits of Blue Light Acne Treatment

Blue light acne treatment focuses on eliminating P. acnes, the bacteria that causes to acne eruptions. These bacteria pumps out some molecules called porphyrins. When these molecules are exposed to blue light, they release free radicals that kill the bacteria.

Blue light acne treatment has several benefits in comparison to other therapies:

- It is a totally natural and has no side effects.

- It is safe to use daily and for all ages.

- Unlike other light therapies, it doesn't contain UV light that can hurt your skin.

- It is painless and you can do it in your own home.

Research Data

Data from clinical trials on blue light therapy has revealed that is a promising acne treatment. Patients involved in the studies have received the blue light acne treatment in several sessions, each lasting about 15 minutes. Many of them, but not all, have registered significant improvement after the treatment, with approximately 55% clearance. Side effects were only mild and included short-term pigment changes, dryness and swelling of the treated area.

Taiwan: Thirty-one patients with facial acne on both sides have received blue light acne treatment only on one side, while the other has received no treatment at all. The therapy was given twice a week for four weeks. In the end, it was concluded that blue light acne treatment is effective unless the patient suffers from cystic acne, which often worsens when treated with blue light.

United States: Twenty-five patients suffering from inflammatory acne were treated with blue light therapy on one side (8 sessions in 4 weeks) and with clindamycin on the other (twice a day for 4 weeks). In the end, researchers compared the results for the two treatments. The side treated with clindamycin showed an approximately 22% improvement, while the one treated with blue light therapy showed around 40% improvement. However, after 8 weeks of no treatment, the clindamycin side had maintained the results better.

Israel: Three separate studies on 10, 13 and 25 patients suffering from inflammatory acne were conducted in order to measure the effects of blue light acne treatment. In all of the three studies, over 80% of all patients responded well to the treatment, showing between 59% and 67% improvement.

Japan: 30 patients suffering from mild to moderate acne received a blue light acne treatment twice a week for up to five weeks. For 80% of all patients, the lesions decreased by approximately 64%. The rest of them experienced negative or no effects.

Unfortunately, the number of individuals involved in these research studies is too small. Generally, clinical trials aimed to test new treatments enroll hundreds or even thousands of patients. Considering the small numbers involved in the blue light acne treatment studies, no statistically valid conclusion can be drawn. However, these studies do reveal that blue light therapy has positive effects on some individuals suffering from acne. It gives best results for inflammatory acne and may not be safe to use on patients with cystic acne lesions.

Chapter 5- Keeping a Clear, Acne-Free Skin

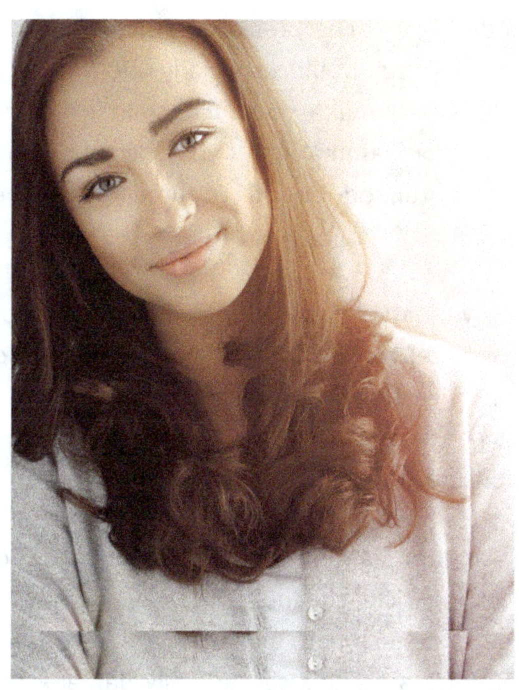

Having acne is an embarrassing prospect for many people. Finding a way to treat it for your specific needs can be difficult. Once you find a way to treat and cure it, acne can be more manageable and easier to maintain. This article can help you find a way to treat acne.

Look for a moisturizer that contains salicylic acid, benzoyl peroxide or retinol. Not only should you make sure your moisturizer is water based, you should also make sure that it combats acne. There are quite a few moisturizers on the market, right now, that contain several useful acne fighting ingredients.

Acne is a skin condition that can cause a lot of embarrassment. Keeping your skin clean will help to reduce the possibility of its occurrence. Use a natural-based cleanser and don't wear a lot of makeup. Keeping your skin clean will allow your pores to breathe and not to get clogged.

Avoid the sun during an acne breakout. The sun can damage your skin in many ways. You should especially avoid it during an acne breakout. Sunlight can make your acne much worse, increasing redness and causing inflammation. If you absolutely must be out in the sun for an extended period of time, remember to wear sunscreen.

For an inexpensive, natural way to help with acne problems, check out what witch hazel can do for you. It contains antioxidant and astringent properties that are effective against acne. Used as an astringent, it is gentle and does not dry out the skin as many other acne medications do.

Consider a moisturizer treatment gel that is designed to moisturize the skin as well as clear acne. There are many moisturizers specifically created to deal with acne. Be careful with products that exfoliate though, because this can actually damage the skin. Find one that is designed to soothe acne symptoms while moisturizing.

An important tip to consider when concerning acne is knowing where acne can occur on your body. This is important in order to distinguish acne from other ailments. Acne will commonly occur on your face, and other times it may show up on the neck, chest, back, or your shoulders. It technically can occur in other places that may have clogged pores, but this would be more likely to occur from bad hygiene.

A great way to help you get rid of acne is to pour a few drops of hydrogen peroxide right on your pimple or affected area. Hydrogen peroxide helps get rid of acne by drying it out. Your acne will be much less noticeable because there will be no bump.

In order to help defeat acne, make sure that your diet consists of a variety of fruits and vegetables. A good diet will give your skin the nutrition/essentials that it needs to help ward off acne and other blemishes from appearing. Try eating a salad once a day or at least having a healthy fruit smoothie.

Using the methods described in this article, you will be able to find a way to treat and cure your acne. These tips will give you ways to keep your skin acne free, but you have to make sure to stick to the skin care regimen tailored to your needs.

Skin Care for the Acne-Prone

When it comes to acne, a lot of information is available from different sources. Old wives' tales, random experiments, and even misguided practices that promise instant cures for acne are followed by many in the hopes of being pimple-free. Unfortunately, some, if not all, of these are without scientific basis and can even make acne worse. Serious skin care for acne-prone skin starts with the right and proper information.

On cures for acne

If myths on the probable causes of acne are abundant, there are also many so-called cures that promise instant freedom from acne. These are:

• Frequent face washing

Since excess oil and dirt are among the causes of acne, some people have this misguided notion that frequently washing one's face can prevent and treat acne. However, this is not the case. Doing so only worsens acne since the skin is stripped off protective lipids which can make it sensitive, dry, and prone to irritations.

• Toothpaste

Toothpaste has antiseptic properties which can cause a pimple to dry out. However, while applying toothpaste to acne may be effective to some, it can cause greater damage to others especially if applied for over time. Toothpaste can dry out surrounding areas and "burn" pimple spots which can lead to discolorations.

• Sun exposure

Probably one of the most idiotic acne myths to surface, some people swear by this. However, sun exposure can only lead to one thing: skin damage. Tans and darker skin tones only hide or camouflage acne but a closer look and touch will reveal bumps and zits. This can make the acne situation worse since sun exposure can make one's skin dry, flaky, discolored, and extra-sensitive.

Eating a balanced diet, exercising, getting enough rest, and following a skin care regimen specific to one's skin type are essential for serious skin care of acne-prone skin. Medications and treatments prescribed by a dermatologist can also help greatly.

Can Acne Cleansers and Lotions Protect Your Skin?

Acne is a common skin disease affecting almost everyone. Acne is caused due to the blockage of skin follicle duct of sebum glands. This blockage traps sebum and causes inflammation of the skin. A bacterium P.Acnes readily infects this inflammation causing acne. There are many common acne products available in the market for acne treatment.

Acne cleansers are facial care products designed to remove dead cells, open up pores, and remove oil, dust, dirt and other harmful pollutants. Generally acne cleansers are used twice or thrice daily and in conjunction with skin toners and moisturizers. Acne cleansers work better than ordinary soap because soap has a very high pH value which can change the pH balance of the skin. The method to use acne cleansers is to use lukewarm water to clean the face then apply acne cleanser all over the face and throat. Next it is to be washed with lukewarm water and then patted dry.

Acne lotions are oil and water emulsions designed to be applied on unbroken skin. Acne lotions are usually medicated with acne medicines like, antibacterial, skin exfoliants, retinoids or antibiotics. Acne lotions may contain soothing or protective ingredients also. Acne lotions have the advantage over creams or ointments as they can be applied thinly over a large area and hence can be economical.

Acne creams are semi solid emulsions. Creams can be used as a barrier for protection, as a delivery vehicle for anti-acne agents and to retain moisture in the skin. Acne cream ingredients may include anti acne agents, moisturizers, skin exfoliants etc.

Acne soaps are mild soaps used to open up the pores and remove oil in excessively oily skins.

All the above products if used in conjunction with acne dietary supplements like Acuzine produce good results. Acuzine consists of anti-oxidants, vitamins E & C, hydrolyzed collagen, ALA, DMAE, Aloe Vera, Bioperine etc. The presence of these ingredients helps in early recovery of the skin and provides vital vitamins and enzymes for rebuilding the skin. Acuzine is available in the form of capsules.

Intrinsic Treatment

The acne skin care industry is a multi-billion dollar industry. Most of the acne clear up products is available through prescription in the industry.

That is the prescription medications for acne are pretty expensive. If you are someone who think who cannot purchase those heavily marketed expensive prescription medications for acne, you should try the alternative medication for acne.

Alternative medication for acne is an intrinsic or natural method for acne treatment. There are many intrinsic products for treating acne. Though they are indeed low in number as compared to the prescription medications, but they have worked for thousands of people.

Many people even don't consider purchasing prescription medications for acne; even they can easily purchase the world-wide marketed prescription medicines without even a fraction of influence on their budgets.

Those people, to avoid getting the harsh side effects of the prescription medicines for acne treatment, come to the alternative means.

So, you should not be disheartened when coming to the intrinsic acne treatments. A lot of the rich and famous people invest their money in intrinsic acne treatment medicines.

Benefits of Intrinsic Acne Treatment:

Following are some of the benefits associated with intrinsic acne treatment that attract masses:

- One Hundred Percent Safe

- Highly Effective

- Low Cost

- Easy Availability

- Ease of Use

Another benefit of using intrinsic acne treatment products is that they are very effective for removing acne scars as well.

You gain everything and lose nothing with intrinsic acne treatment.

Chapter 6- Acne Leaves Marks

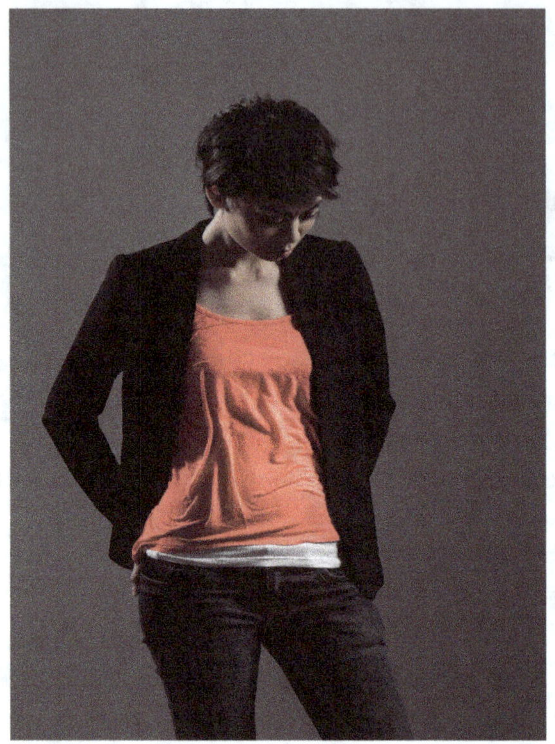

With some ailments, the name says it all. Acne, the dreaded symptom that manifests itself as pimples or zits, is scientifically called Acne vulgaris. And true to its name, it is unsightly and often causes more than physical scarring among millions of teens worldwide. But like any other bodily manifestation, acne too has a cure.

Sure, there are a wide array of them available in the marketplace to help you choose from, but truth be told, acne is not a permanent condition and acne cures that work actually exist.

Before one starts looking at available acne cures, it might be a good idea to try and understand what causes acne in the first place. Contrary to popular belief, acne is not caused by bad facial hygiene.

Nearly everyone believes this though and any acne cures, which stem from this belief, are unlikely to work. What cause acne however are hormonal changes in the body that result in the production of excessive oil from the sebaceous glands.

In some other cases, acne is caused when the pores are blocked or when the sebaceous glad itself is a victim of some infection. In order to work, acne cures must first target the underlying problem.

An acne cure that targets the infection of the sebaceous glad for instance is unlikely to work in a case when the acne is a direct result of hair duct blockage. Like with any other illness, acne cures too must target and work on the root cause of the problem.

There are several kinds of acne cures available in the market. First, there are topical acne cures. These usually comprise some creams or lotions that can be applied directly to the affected area.

These kinds of acne cures normally include topical antibiotics, glycolic acid, lactic acid and gluconic acid. In some cases, such acne cures might also involve an active ingredient like azelaic acid cream and in cases where the acne is severe, Accutane and sotret might be active components.

Apart from the topical, there are also several oral acne cures available. Most chemists and drugstores have a wide variety of oral acne cures available readily on their shelves.

However, before using such acne cures, it might be a good idea to see a dermatologist, who can not only identify the cause of your individual acne, but also prescribe the most suitable treatment for you.

A recent innovation in the acne research field has brought to the fore another kind of acne cure. This is laser acne treatment and is becoming increasingly popular as the results have proven to be spectacular.

It's nothing to be Embarrassed About!

Adult Acne is not something to feel embarrassed about. Though the general notion is that acne and pimple outbreaks are for pre-pubertal and teenaged populations, adult acne is not unusual. A majority of adults, who were lucky to be 'acne free' during their teenage years and who saw the desperation of their peers trying to combat acne, feel mortified when they find that just when they assumed they were free of acne forever, they have become afflicted by adult acne.

Most of the adults are confused and embarrassed. They wonder, isn't acne an adolescent problem? But the truth remains that adult acne is more widespread than imagined. Statistics show that in the United States alone, nearly 40% of all acne cure products are purchased and used by adult acne sufferers.

What is the reason behind adult acne? Well. It is not one but many. However, the most universally attributed cause, that of bad personal hygiene, is a myth. Nearly all acne cases even adult acne, are a direct consequence of blocked pores on the skin or hormonal imbalances. Faulty closing of facial hair ducts or infection of the oil glands are a probable cause of adult acne.

The good news is that acne can be cured to a greater or lesser degree. The bad news is that most adults, in their zeal to overcome the embarrassment of an adult acne outbreak, try the first remedy they can lay their hands on from their neighborhood drugstore. Little do they think that this could do more harm than good to their acne problem. The remedies found over the counter cater to acne problems of the majority of the younger populations. These medications and remedies might not have the potency or the capacity to deal with adult acne because the reasons of which may vary to a great degree.

Adult acne demands tougher remedies despite the fact that adult acne is no different from regular acne. So what should be the first step to cure adult acne? A good idea is to consult the dermatologist to determine the underlying cause of what caused adult acne. The next step after the diagnosis is done is to use simple prescription drugs to eradicate the acne problem forever.

However, there is one important piece of advice. All adult acne sufferers need not be embarrassed about their problem. Like I stated above, adult acne is commoner than imagined. So which option do you feel is better? To make that one visit to the dermatologist to do away with your acne problem or to spend a fortune at the local pharmacist in trying to find the elixir for acne in addition to the fear and worry that comes with it? Think about it. The choice is yours.

About the Author

Janet Crawford is a dermatologist. She has seen patients complaining of mild to severe acne. Most of them, according to Janet, have very low self-esteem. As a professional, Janet has a deep understanding on many skin conditions and their underlying reasons that's why she feels sad that many would have to face issues with their self-worth when it couldn't have been the case.

In 2012, Janet launched a campaign to spread awareness on acne. The goal is to empower patients to live seek help and keep their self-esteem high while they're struggling with the disease.

At present, Janet is a known voice in the subject and is often sought for help in their local community.

www.ingramcontent.com/pod-product-compliance
Lightning Source LLC
Chambersburg PA
CBHW050705250726
48662CB00002B/857